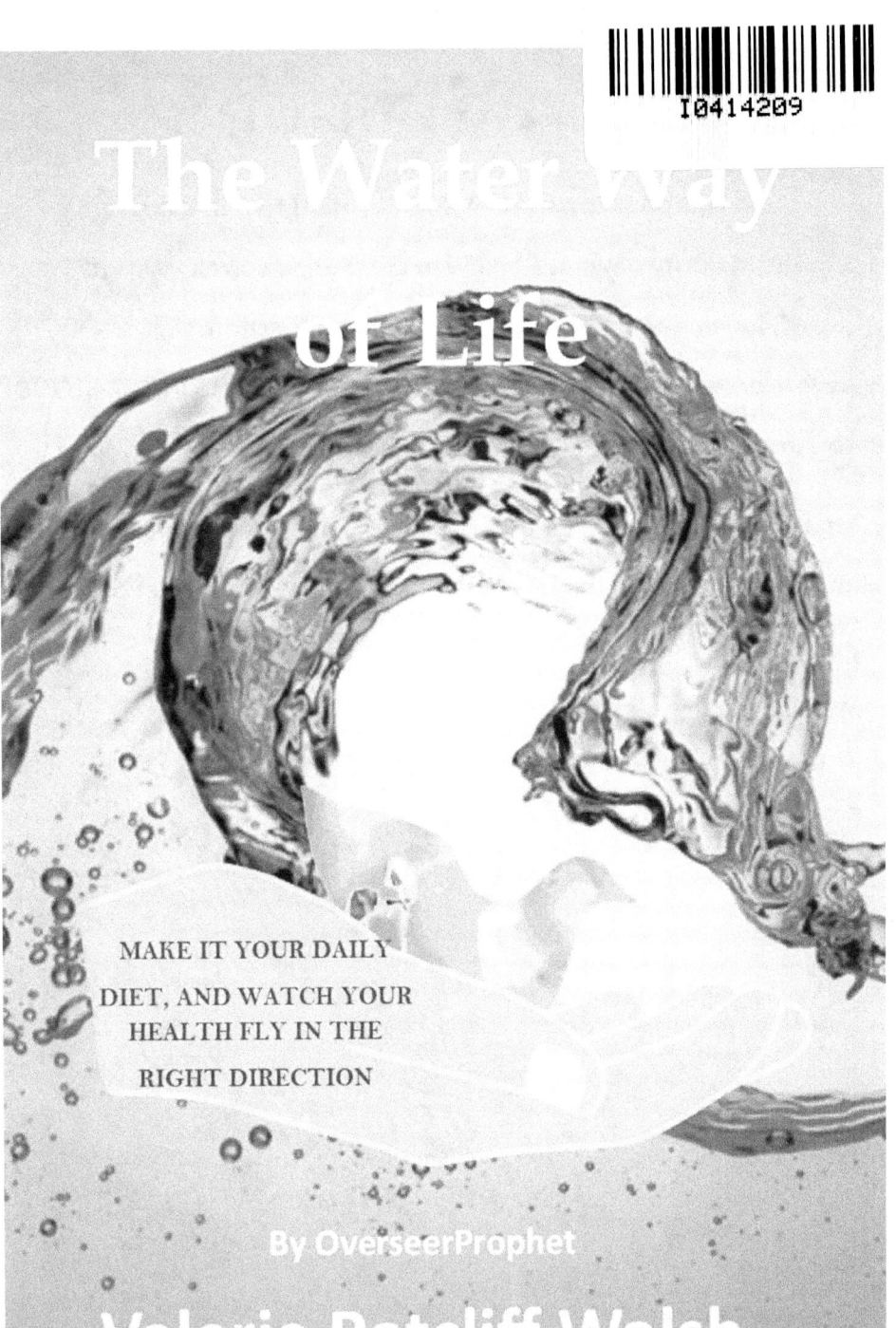

The Water Way of Life

MAKE IT YOUR DAILY
DIET, AND WATCH YOUR
HEALTH FLY IN THE
RIGHT DIRECTION

By OverseerProphet

Valerie Ratcliff Walsh

© Copyright 2016, The Water Way of Life, Valerie Ratcliff Walsh, All Rights Reserved

Introduction

This book is part of my GODLY HEALTH SERIES.

The majority of what God did in creation, involved WATER!

And, he made the majority of our body to function off WATER!

Believe it or Not, THERE IS LIFE IN WATER, AS THE LIFE IS IN THE BLOOD!

In this book, there are five (5) Water campaigns available for you to try. You can start at the beginners, or you can go straight for the big one. It's all up to you. But, whatever you do, you need to drink water.

I'm going to talk a whole lot about water to you. When I get through, we are going to go on a campaign together. We are going to win for ourselves and then help others win too.

I PRAY YOU ENJOY IT, AND FOLLOW THE INSTRUCTIONS GOD HAS GIVEN ME, WITH EXPERIENCE, TO GIVE TO YOU.

INSTRUCTIONS

THROUGH MUCH PRAYER AND GODLY DIRECTION, I AM LED TO WRITE, PUBLISH AND DISTRIBUTE MY BOOK ON WATER.

PLEASE PRAY BEFORE USING THESE DIRECTIONS AND PLEASE CONSULT A DOCTOR BEFORE IMPLEMENTING MY INSTRUCTIONS.

IN ADDITION, IF YOU HAVE ANY HEALTH ISSUES, ASK YOUR DOCTOR IF YOU MAY USE THIS WATER GUIDE IN WHOLE OR IN PART.

TAKE THIS BOOK TO YOUR DOCTOR AND LET THEM KNOW YOU'VE BEEN READING IT.

DISCLOSURE

I, MY BUSINESS, MINISTRIES OR ANY ASSOCIATIONS I HAVE, ARE NOT RESPONSIBLE FOR ANY SIDE EFFECTS OR ANY CAUSES AND EFFECTS, FOR YOUR USE OR FOLLOWING THE INSTRUCTIONS IN THIS WATER BOOK. MY SEMINARS OR PRODUCTS AND SERVICES IN WHOLE OR IN PART ARE EXEMPT FROM ANY LIABILITY, LOSS, DAMAGES, ETC. WATER IS A NATURAL FLUID AND IS NOT HARMFUL ON IT'S OWN UNDER NORMAL CIRCUMSTANCES. YOU ARE INSTRUCTED TO CONSULT YOUR OWN DOCTOR BEFORE USING AND IMPLEMENTING THE ADVICE AND INSTRUCTIONS IN THIS MANUAL.

WATER – H2O

2 Hydrogen

1 Oxygen

Water is a transparent fluid which forms the world's streams, lakes, oceans and rain, and is the major constituent of the fluids of organisms. As a chemical compound, a water molecule contains one oxygen and two hydrogen atoms that are connected by covalent bonds.

Water (H_2O) is the most abundant compound on Earth's surface, covering 70 percent of the planet. In nature, water exists in liquid, solid, and gaseous states. It is in dynamic equilibrium between the liquid and gas states at standard temperature and pressure. At room temperature, it is a tasteless and odorless liquid, nearly colorless with a hint of blue. Many substances dissolve in water and it is commonly referred to as the universal solvent. Because of this, water in nature and in use is rarely pure and some properties may vary from those of the pure substance. However, there are also many compounds that are essentially, if not completely, insoluble in water. Water is the only common substance found naturally in all three common states of matter and it is essential for all life on Earth. Water makes up 55% to 78% of the human body.

YOUR BODY NEEDS WATER TO SURVIVE. AND, IF YOU DON'T GET ENOUGH WATER, YOU WILL GET SICK AND DIE. YOU WILL DRY UP LIE A RAISIN AND LOOK TERRIBLE BEFORE YOU EXPIRE.

FIVE BENEFITS TO DRINKING WATER:

1.) Supports metabolism

Water helps keeps your metabolic rate up (cellular hydration is necessary for cellular metabolism); allows you to tell whether you're really hungry or just thirsty (you can mistake hunger for thirst), and has no sugar or artificial sweeteners (you're keeping it natural – what your body likes).

2.) Promotes vitality

Dehydration can cause tired eyes, headaches, and a case of the "blahs." Drinking enough water helps promote your wellbeing. And remember, by the time you're thirsty, you're dehydrated. Keep it flowing throughout the day!

3.) Helps with digestion

Staying hydrated keeps things moving along smoothly in your digestive tract. Water is necessary to breakdown your food and prevent constipation.

4.) Eliminates toxins

Water helps your kidneys flush out toxins you don't need in your system through urination. Sweat is another natural way your body removes waste products – drink up!

5.) Improves muscle strength

Muscles need hydration too! When muscles have enough fluid, they can work longer and harder, helping you get stronger and have more energy – and who doesn't want that?

Where did Water come from?

Water came from GOD. Believe it or not. It is one of the Natural elements of God. God created all of the elements and they work on his behalf and by his glorious power. These elements have the attributes of GOD.

WATER IS GOD'S MOVING WAY. WATER MOVES JUST LIKE GOD.

Water is Patient and flows freely to bless you. All of God's elements are in his control. God made them all. They didn't just appear. God CREATED EVERYTHING.

All things that were made, were made by him. And, without him was NOT anything made that was made. UNDERSTAND? Good.

In the first book of the Bible, Genesis, God divides the waters. Obviously water was covering everything. The water he divided and moved, left dry land to appear which is now called Earth. He made seas and then because the dry land had already been watered, he called forth grass, herb, yielding seed, fruit tree, yielding fruit after his kind, whose seed is in itself, upon the earth: and it was so.

God created us out of the dust of the Earth. We are earthlings. We are created by God.

Our bodies are actually self-sufficient when given our proper yielding seed after our kind. Along with Water, our body will yield more of the fruit that we need to endure rather than, that which causes adverse consequences to our health, strength and longevity.

What does water do?

Water Cleanses. Water moves things. Water settles things. Water secures things. Water moisturizes. Water loosens. Water pushes things deeper. Water divides. Water evens things. Water dilutes. Water not only creates foundations, Water helps make a soluble foundation for ingestion and digestion. Water makes things grow. Water blesses the blood. The blood is our life………….

But most importantly, water takes flight. I'm sure you will exclaim, What? Are you saying that water can fly? Well, maybe not fly. But, it can rise to the sky. And, in rising, it always lifts up and saves. It may not fly. But it does take flight. Let me explain the difference.

Something that can fly, probably has natural wings. It can literally and physically fly up into the sky and maintain itself by flapping with God given precision and at rapid speed, soaring and gliding. But, that which doesn't have wings can still fly by taking flight, and able to maintain itself by power and substance. Wings are created by other greatness and rareness aside from being physically attached. If there is enough power pushing it, water can fly. Water will clear it up, fix it up and save it.

When water enters your body, it immediately, with great speed and precision (if I may), begins to hydrate and revive any and all parts in need. It quickens and blesses the organs and helps with blood flow. And, you even need water for your bones. You want your entire body to stay moist, flexible and easy moving! It's called Hydration. This means your body has the required amount or enough water to function easily and properly.

The opposite of hydration is dehydration. This means your body is dried out or in the process of drying out. Dehydrated – Already dried out or in the process of drying out. Dehydration – Going through the process of drying out. Either one is dangerous.

*********A LACK OF DRINKING WATER, DETERIORATES THE HUMAN BODY*********

These are some of `the effects of dehydration:

High Blood Pressure

Heart Problems

High Blood Sugar

Fatigue

Joint problems

Stiffness

Arthritis

Skin Disorders

Asthma and Allergies

High Cholesterol

Bladder and Kidney problems

Digestive disorders

And more!

Why? You may ask. Because your organs are overworking and your body is not functioning properly. Everything is going haywire and malfunctioning. Like a plane that has stopped working and one of the wings are gone, you are headed for a hard landing (CRASH!) that you may not survive. And, if you are in the heat (Hot Weather) at the same time, you may not be conscious when you crash.

No matter what Faith, Religion, Race, Creed, Color, National Origin, Marital Status, Preferences or whatever else you can think of:

YOU NEED TO DRINK WATER!

GOD WANTS YOU TO DRINK WATER

YOUR BODY WANTS YOU TO DRINK WATER

EVERYBODY ON EARTH, NEEDS TO DRINK WATER

When one is dehydrated, there is an absence of water and moisture in the body. Your body cannot function as it should. And your body is not functioning properly without your knowledge. You will receive warnings only when your body is so dehydrated, your skin and lips crack, your urine is yellow or your organs are becoming weak and are starting to dysfunction. Unless you are a person who is always hydrated, then, you may get warning signs quicker because your body may immediately tell you that it is not getting its normal dose. Isn't that funny. A body that is always being neglected of hydration, seems to work in stages. It will eventually sneak up on you. But, the consequences may be great and unrecoverable. But a healthy body, gives warnings a lot sooner. Why? Because it will immediately crave what it is accustomed to. So, your warning signs will kick in sooner than later. GOOD HEALTH IS ALWAYS ON TOP. GOOD HEALTH WARNS SOONER AND HAS AN EASIER AND BETTER CHANCE OF PREVENTION AND RECUPERATION.

Directed to Water

When I was a kid, my youngest brother and I use to have water contests. We would drink so much water until our stomachs would swell up. LOL One day, my brother and I drank so much water, we fell asleep. Our mother was worried to say the least. But we were fine. We were just so silly; back then. LOL

We always had clear skin and always got a clean bill of health at the Doctor's office.

Our parents never had a problem with us drinking water. Both my Mom and Dad were water drinkers. No Soda, limited sweet drinks and always juice and milk. If we had soda, it was for a special occasion or something. To this day, Soda is just too strong for me. I drink a little once in a while. But, it is not my thing, THANK GOD.

At breakfast, we always had, Juice, milk and water with a full healthy meal.

Anyway, for some reason, we all seemed to love water. People would think we were strange, because we would drink water and actually think that water tastes good. To this day, we all still like water and still think it tastes good. We all like milk too. LOL

But, we love water. Maybe because it's so refreshing and thirst quenching. Or, maybe because it's so smooth and goes down easy. Could it be because when it's cold, it cools the entire body? Especially in the summertime. Most likely, it's probably because we were taught to drink it from a very young age and we acquired a taste for it. Hint, Hint.

I remember at Church, one of my older sisters and I would talk to friends about drinking water. They would absolutely hate water. Many of them would say that it tastes nasty and that they couldn't stand to drink it. Most of them were also soda and fruit punch drinkers. Fruit punch was a big deal then. So was KOOL-AID. Yuk, I absolutely hate Kool-Aid and I always refused to drink it. Of course, I was called stuck up because of it. No, I just hate it. It tastes like colored water no matter how much sugar you put in it. And, the more sugar you put in it, the nastier it tastes. I CAN'T EVEN TELL YOU, HOW MUCH I HATE KOOL-AID. Ok, back to water. I was having a moment there. So, even at school, kids didn't drink a lot of water. And many would say that they didn't drink it at home either. Those who brought snacks or lunch to school would have bags loaded with sodas and sweet drinks. And, lots of junk foods too.

Here's what is so funny. Those same people wouldn't like orange juice or milk either. They also hated cheese and fruit. I always found that odd. But, Don't get too happy if you are juice and milk drinkers either. Orange Juice and Milk are not what they use to be. You've got to be careful with the sweet juices and the fat in the milk.

So, I realize that in order for adults to drink and like to drink water, they probably need to be taught from a baby or childhood to drink and like water. They will acquire a taste for it with or without understanding its benefits.

My mother and father used to tell us the benefits of water. But, when you are a kid. You do it, because you were told to. When you become an adult, you do it because you actually understand it. Either you look and feel great because of it, you had a bad experience that taught you to finally do what you've been taught, or you just didn't know in the first place.

My parents were southern people, so they would easily tell you that you would die without it. Which is true. But, the way they said it, was like you would die right then and there, if you didn't hurry up and get some water. That's the southern way. Old wives tales and scaring you half to death to get you to do something. LOL But, They did it in a fun way. We were keen kids, just like them. So, we knew we wouldn't die right then and there. But, just to play along, please them, and because they made it so much fun, we would get some yummy water and drink it up. They would drink it themselves and say how good it tastes. Of course, we wanted to be like mommy and daddy, so, we drank the water and said it tasted good too.

The point I'm trying to make is that we were simply directed to water. Like anything else, if you point your children to water, they will drink it. Be the example and drink it yourself. Don't give me the do as I say, not as I do, line. That one has failed in every other area, and is not about to start working now. You can bring a child to water and you can make them drink, but it's better to be a good example and have them imitate you. You probably should start from when they are first born. A yummy bottle full of water. Yippie! Let them acquire a taste for it. Then, all of you are good to go.

But, what if you are an adult who doesn't like water. Refuse to drink water and think it's never gonna catch up with you. Hopefully, you don't have children whom you are teaching the same destructive behavior. Because, to get southern on you, that's a death sentence for you and all of yours. BIG MISTAKE.

Well, I'm here to Direct you to water. You can teach your kids and your kids will teach their kids and so on.

Direct your kids to water. They will Direct their kids to water and you will all be going in the right direction to find the WATER WAY OF LIFE.

We are eating too much!

One of my older sister's and I were NOT big eaters when we were younger. We would eat enough, but we had a very high metabolism and wouldn't gain a pound. Like I said before. We were very healthy and always got a clean bill of health at the Doctor. We were very active children. Happy, jumping around, running, playing and having lots of fun.

So, as you can see, the kids today already have a problem because they are always in the house or playing with gadgets. You hardly ever see kids taking off running and losing their minds in laughter and play.

They go from eating to texting, to eating to video games, to eating to movies, to eating to youtube, to eating back to texting, to eating to staring at something again and back to eating. And, electronics from some reason, make you want to snack and eat. So, if you are on them all the time, you are probably eating all the time.

But, even those who don't stay on phones, tablets and Tv's all the time are still eating too much. And, they are eating junk. Flavorful, delicious, loaded with Salt and Sugar, JUNK. Remember: If it's not home cooked or homemade style, IT'S FAST FOOD!

Whatever they put in the food to get us addicted is just plain old WRONG. Everywhere you go, people are over eating and getting bigger and Bigger and BIGGER!

A body overstuffed and overly full needs more water to break it up and disperse its nutrients in the right directions, as well as excrete what is unwanted and unnecessary.

You may laugh. But, I believe there is an adverse spirit of OVER EATING loose in the world. IT'S CALLED GLUTTONY. Not just with food. But we are "OVER-INTAKING" in too many areas of our lives. FOOD JUST HAPPENS TO BE THE BIG ONE THAT MORE IMMEDIATELY, CAUSES ADVERSE RESULTS.

BUT WE ARE USING TOO MANY DEVICES, TOO MANY HOURS A DAY. WE ARE OVER PURCHASING, OVER ENGAGING AND JUST OVER DOING IT ALTOGETHER. SHAME ON US ALL.

This has got to change.

The rich used to suffer alone concerning access to too much and too many things. They were still unhappy. But, now everybody is in the running for overdoing everything and suffering the consequences. THE RICH LIFE HAS COME AND RUINED A LOT OF PEOPLE. YOU DON'T HAVE TO BE RICH TO LIVE A RICH LIFE ANYMORE. And, I truly believe that those who want to offer us more for less have the best intentions at first. However, when they realize that this "OVER-ACCESS" is ruining our children, our congregations, our people and our country, THE MEANS FROM THE GAINS CLOUD THEIR JUDGMENT AND THEY REFUSE TO CARE. If they had the heart to do something good from the beginning, it's still in there somewhere. But, they have covered it with stones. And, now they have stony hearts.

But, this behavior from ourselves and others have great consequences in the long run.

WE HAVE GOT TO STOP, AND STOP NOW.

I WANT YOU TO GO ON THE REVERSAL CAMPAIGN WITH ME. YOU WILL FIND THAT CAMPAIGN IN MY OTHER BOOK WHICH IS A PART OF THIS "GODLY HEALTH SERIES".

So, back to food. Food is intended for you to nourish, maintain and continue living. IT IS A NECESSITY, NOT A LUXURY. Although, in some places to all of our SHAME, it is a luxury for some. A luxury in the reverse sense that they only time some people get food is on very special occasions. We need to feed the hungry people. I MUST INCLUDE COMMENTS OF CONSCIOUSNESS AT ALL TIMES. It is important for us to always be mindful of others who are suffering, while we sit up and freely write about what is right and wrong and what must be done. While others have no such options. We must be grateful for our opportunities and Blessings from God. And, as we better ourselves, let us NOT forget to reach out and help others. GOD BLESS YOU.

Now, WE ARE EATING TOO MUCH. We are loading it in everyday, all day. There is a reason why nutritionist and doctors always talked about three full meals a day or five to six small meals a day. THAT IS NOT HOW WE ARE LIVING TODAY!

ONE MEAL IS LIKE TWO FULL MEALS, PLUS DESSERT, PLUS SWEET DRINKS, PLUS MORE AND MORE AND MORE.

IT IS A SIGN OF UNHAPPINESS AND COVERING UP.

This overeating and doing things adverse to our well being is a sign that the world in general, is in hiding mode, instead of dealing and resolving anymore.

It shows up in every area of government, industry and individuals.

LIVE A LIFE THAT IS OUT OF CONTROL, UNREPENTANT, UNFORGIVING, ANGRY, CARELESS, CALOUS, FOOLISH, OUTRAGEOUS, FAST PACED AND WITHOUTH THOUGHT. THEN, PUT A BANDAID ON IT WHEN IT GETS BROKEN OR SCARRED, AND THEN BLOW IT UP OR CUT IT; IF THAT DOESN'T WORK.

FIND ANY OTHER SOLUTION EXCEPT THE RIGHT ONE. DISCOVERY, ACKNOWLEDGMENT, ACCEPTANCE, CHANGE & DISCIPLINE.

But, because we are eating too much and NOT DRINKING WATER, we are tired and not thinking straight enough to follow any steps to doing better.

THAT'S WHY I WROTE THIS BOOK. AND I AM ON THIS CAMPAIGN TRAIL MYSELF AND INVITE EVERYBODY IN THE WORLD TO GO ON IT WITH ME.

We've got to change our diets.

First we have already discovered through MY BOOK (SMILE), countless health reports, doctor's findings and warnings and news stories, about how the world is over eating and causing harm to ourselves. THAT IS DISCOVERY.

Now, we must ACKNOWLEDGE that we are doing the wrong thing and start doing the right thing, right now.

ACCEPT the fact that you have to change and have to grow up. Accept the remedies offered and given to you to do better. THIS IS ACCEPTANCE.

Make a CHANGE immediately. This change will save your life and others you are responsible for. It will also touch the lives of others who see you change.

DISCIPLINE YOUR SELF. Teach yourself and practice how to do right. You will become accustomed to doing what is good and beneficial for you.

LIFE IS MORE THAN FOOD! WE ARE EATING TOO MUCH! GOD IS NOT PLEASED! WE HAVE BECOME GLUTTONS!

Drop the utensil, Push away from the table, back away from the kitchen and tell yourself. I will not defile my body anymore and have God destroy it. No more overdoing it. Take what you need and save the rest for another day. PORTIONS. It's not just a word.

Get rid of Salt and Sugar!

This is a warning! **Get rid of added Salt and Sugar completely. And stay away from salty and sugary foods altogether. God will give you the Water Way of Life if you will not dry your body out with Salt and Sugar.**

Salt and Sugar are a big mess. I will not separate them because they are both VERY HARMFUL. One is not less harmful than the other. If you let them, and fall into their trap, If Salt doesn't get you, Sugar will. If Sugar doesn't get you, Salt will. THEY ARE A GANG OF THUGS LOOKING TO ROB AND KILL YOU.

Salt and Sugar dries you out. Salt sucks up all the water out of your body and SO DOES SUGAR. Sugar is just as much of a destroyer as Salt. Hurtful to the organs and the entire body. Both of them are like DRUGS. Destroying your thought patterns, putting you on a high and taking your moods and feelings up and down EVERY time you injest, too much of them. When a person is severely diabetic and they don't have their insulin, they are told to drink a lot of water. It will keep their blood sugar down until they get their insulin. If they are diabetic, they will still need their medication. But, Water MAY help fight off fainting or going into a coma. But, it is not a cure for diabetes. But, certainly a PREVENTION to diabetes. Also cinnamon can significantly lower your blood sugar. However, taking cinnamon with insulin medication can lower your blood sugar to the extreme. PLEASE: ASK YOUR DOCTOR FIRST.

Drinking Water can lower blood sugar levels by diluting the amount of glucose(sugar) in the blood stream. Indirectly, it will reduce insulin resistance and help a person reduce their hunger. So, Drinking water lowers blood sugar and makes you less hungry. It leaves you less room to consume out of your lust for food. And, if you have a problem with loving salt and sugar, it will keep you from eating too much of it. BECAUSE YOUR STOMACH IS FULL. If you want to do better and live. Here is your opportunity in this book.

Back to Salt. Salt is a quick and calculating killer and we all better watch ourselves. There is supposed to be just enough salt in your food to make it taste good. But, you need to add different spices and ingredients to make it taste good. NOT POUR A BOX OF SALT ON IT TO GET TASTE AND END UP EATING A SALT MEAL. You are supposed to be able to taste the flavor of the meat or food that you are eating. Each food has its own flavor. All you want to do is enhance. Not kill the thing, TWICE. Once you load it with too much salt, you can't get any nutrients out of it. It's like drinking a box of salt. You wasted your time cooking or eating because you destroyed the purpose of the food. NOURISHMENT!

High Blood Pressure and High Blood Sugar are some of the worse conditions you can have. PLEASE WORK AT STAYING HEALTHY OR REVERSE YOUR CURRENT CONDITIONS.

YOU DO NOT NEED ADDED SALT OR SUGAR. You only need a VERY little of both. SHAME ON ALL OF US FOR DEFILING OUR

BODIES. REPENT TO GOD AND DO BETTER TO THE SAVING OF YOUR OWN LIFE.

TAKE CARE OF YOUR SKIN!

Along with water, take care of your skin. Your skin will automatically begin to shine with a good diet and lots of water. However, your skin must still be moisturized and appetized by good stuff on the outside. Water will clear it up, but you must still keep it up. Vitamin E, Cocoa Butter, Shea Butter and other delicious creams & oils are awesome for the skin.

Water will get rid of the bags under your eyes unless it's just hereditary. And, even then, it won't be as bad as it was before.

Just like you feed your insides to work properly, look good on an x-ray, feel good and work good for you, do the same for your skin. FEED YOUR SKIN NUTRIENTS AND NATURAL PRODUCTS.

Stay away from make-up. The make-up industry is going to be mad at me. But, you are caking up a bunch of junk on your face and it is killing your skin. It just makes you age more, so you can buy more of their mess, to prevent the aging they are causing. Sorry make-up industry. The reason for your make-up is not a problem, as long as you are not trying to fake-up. Meaning, you are not just trying to look good, look better or hide blemishes. You are actually trying to be somebody else. That's not good. Food for thought my friend. Anything you do to yourself, should be for the sole purpose of advancing yourself, and being able to get along in this society.

I understand how you feel. But, love yourself. Don't hate yourself. And, don't think anybody else is greater than you and push yourself to imitate or copy others. Water is a natural skin fixer. Make-up is a temporary concealer.

If you are in the entertainment business, on TV or take pictures and video all the time, or you wear Make-Up for work related or medical reasons, that is your business and your right. I am not talking about you. But, maybe you should get extra insurance (make the industry pay for it or write it off on your taxes) for the side effects or other future problems it could cause.

Your urine should be CLEAR!

If you go to use the bathroom and your urine is yellow. Depending on how yellow, you may be dehydrated. If your urine smells a lot, you are definitely dehydrated and your urine is probably dark. If your urine is very dark or very, very dark, you are severely dehydrated and may need to see a doctor right away.

The Test: If your urine is very dark or very, very dark, Drink two full glasses of water and wait to use the bathroom. If the first time you use the bathroom after drinking the two glasses, your urine is still dark. Repeat the test. Drink two more glasses of water. If the second time you use the bathroom, your urine is still dark. Call the Doctor and make an appointment immediately.

After drinking that much water, your urine should lighten up unless you have some condition that you already know about. Or, you are taking some kind of medication that dehydrates you. In which case, you need to double up on the water to replenish your liquids. If medication is causing your urine to get dark as a side effect. Make sure you inform your doctor and see what the doctor says.

If you ever have black urine, CALL AN AMBULANCE IMMEDIATELY.

Your Urine should be clear and should not have a bad smell.

What will happen when I start to drink more water?

You will look better, feel better, have more energy, be healthy, get a better bill of health unless something else is wrong. But, water can only help every situation unless you have an overworked or bad kidney or some other condition that could have an adverse reaction to water. That's why you should stay in good health and consult a doctor if anything seems wrong.

You will have a softer, easy stool. Meaning you won't be constipated and you will use the bathroom easily.

Your food will digest better and easier. You will be able to get more nutrients out of your "Healthy Meals".

Your skin will be moist and heal easily if you get a cut or something.

Your Hair will shine. Your nails won't be brittle. You won't have dark circles (unless hereditary) and scars & marks will clear up faster.

Brain functions and all organs will work properly or better.

YOU WILL LOOK & FEEL BETTER. YOU WILL BE HEALTHIER. THIS IS MOST IMPORTANT. DRINK YOUR WATER.

Water Campaigns

My water campaigns are easy to start, continue and finish. You just have to be a little dedicated and want to be a whole lot healthy.

This water campaign is based on NOT CONSUMING MORE THAN 8 – 8oz GLASSES OF WATER A DAY. Too much water can overwork the kidneys. That's dangerous and very harmful to your body. 8 -8oz Glasses = Campaign. LET'S GO!

To go on one of my water campaigns, you must take a vow.

VOW

(Say aloud)

1 – I vow to be true to the water campaign and follow the campaign that I choose strictly and properly.

2 – I vow to consult a doctor and get a check-up before I go on this campaign.

3 – I vow to eat fruits and vegetables and healthy foods during and after this campaign.

4 – I vow to exercise as much as I can during and after this campaign.

5 – I vow to complete my campaign and try the next stage if possible.

6 – I vow to take better care of myself from here on.

7 – I vow to do my best.

This campaign is to help you "thin it out"! Plus, it's a little trick to help you want to drink water. When you drink a little juice or something else more desirable before your water, it makes it easier to drink the water, whether you like water or not. Sometimes, when you don't feel like drinking water. Drink a little of something else first, then you will gladly drink the water. It gets easier. That's why Mix & Match is good for beginners. Even children.

When you are on this campaign, I want you to drink a quarter glass of water before every meal and a quarter glass of water after every meal. I want you to mix and match with water and other drinks. Put both water and your beverage on the table before you, and keep switching between them and drinking a little of both until you acquire a taste for water.

This campaign will also help to discourage you from drinking sugary drinks. The combination of the water, beverage mix and match will confuse your taste buds and choose the water every time. You will see. You will begin to want more water than any other beverage. Or, you will at least acquire a taste for water and begin to think that water taste good.

Many people say that water doesn't have a flavor. But, to water lovers, it's sweet like candy and better than any other beverage. I'm going to help you get there.

People who hate water, normally just leave the water in a restaurant on the table or ask for it to be removed. You will be keeping yours or supplying your own. Either way, stick with your campaign.

So, when you are at the dinner table, you should have already drank a quarter glass of water before your meal. Then you should be mixing and matching the exact same amount of water and beverage as you dine. After your meal, you should have another quarter glass of water to end it all.

If you are having a desert afterwards, you must drink another quarter glass of water before and after your desert. Each time, Every time.

If you are drinking a beverage leisurely, you still must mix and match. You can't just buy a beverage without also buying a bottle of water to mix and match with.

All other times during the day, you are sipping water only.

Don't cheat. See your campaign through.

BEGIN AGAIN: 25% Water – This is a campaign for those who just forget to drink water and don't think about how important water is.

This is the campaign to help you become a devout water drinker. When you are on this campaign, you are also drinking a quarter glass of water before and after each meal. However, you are also drinking another quarter glass of water during your meal and only a quarter glass of another beverage during your meal. No more and no less. You are not allowed to drink more than a quarter glass of another beverage during your meal.

At the dinner table or at any meal, you should have already had a quarter glass of water before, a quarter glass of water during, only one quarter glass of another beverage during and a quarter glass of water afterwards.

If you are having dessert, then you must again drink another quarter glass of water before and after that dessert. And, you can only have one quarter glass of water during the dessert and one quarter glass of another beverage during the dessert.

When you are drinking a beverage leisurely, you are drinking a quarter glass of water at the beginning and end of that beverage and no more than fifty percent of the beverage at any given time.

At all other times during the day, you are grabbing a quarter glass of water.

You are drinking more water than other beverages at all times.

PUSH IT: 50% Water – This is the dedicated campaign for water drinkers who still need juices and sodas to get along daily.

This campaign is to boost water drinkers to the next level. When you are on this campaign, you are drinking half a glass of water before and after every meal. You are also drinking half a glass of water during your meal and half a glass of another beverage during your meal.

At the dinner table, you should have already had a half glass of water before your meal, during your meal, a half glass of another beverage and then a half glass of water after your meal.

If you have dessert, you must have half a glass of water before and after the dessert, and no more than half a glass of another beverage during the dessert.

At all other times during the day, you are drinking a half glass of water.

Cutting other beverages as much as possible will benefit you and your body greatly.

OVER THE HUMP: 75% Water – This is the more than enough campaign for lovers of water who still drink other beverages.

This campaign is to encourage you to stay in the race and put on your game face. If you drink this much water, you are at athlete status already and can do whatever activities you want without dehydrating or worrying. But, this also depends on your current health, any conditions and doctor's orders. ☺

When on this campaign, you are drinking a full glass of water 15-30 minutes before a meal. You are drinking only half a glass of another beverage during a meal. You are drinking a half glass of water after your meal.

If you are having dessert, you are drinking a half glass of water before that dessert. You are not drinking anything else with the dessert. If you do, you must drink another half glass of water after the dessert. Then, 15-30 minutes later, you are drinking another half glass of water.

If you are drinking a beverage leisurely, you are drinking a half glass of water and drinking only half a glass of the other beverage. Then you are drinking another half glass of water afterwards. 15-30 minutes later, you are drinking another half glass of water.

At all other times during the day, you are drinking a half glass of water. No other beverages except for hot beverages in between.

You are on your way to the water way!

THE MASTERS: 100% Water – This is the hard charger campaign for health lovers who will take water over everything else and drink other beverages once in a while or once a day.

This campaign is for the WATER WAY OF LIFE! YIPPIE JESUS!

When on this campaign, you are drinking water at all times. You may drink one other beverage a day. But, just one. So choose wisely.

You are drinking a full glass of water at every meal. Even if you are drinking your one other beverage during that meal, you must drink a full glass of water.

You must get 8-8oz glasses of water a day. NOT MORE THAN THAT! However, you may have two hot beverages a day. You are a Master.

You are drinking water at breakfast, lunch and dinner. You are drinking water in between and at ALL TIMES.

YOU ARE IN THE WATER WAY OF LIFE.

You are serious about living longer, living healthy, living whole, living happy, living free and just living in general.

For you, it's all about water and the "THE WATER WAY OF LIFE"!

CHOOSE A CAMPAIGN

Now, choose a campaign and get going to better health and a better life.

I'll be rooting for you and I know God will be pleased with you.

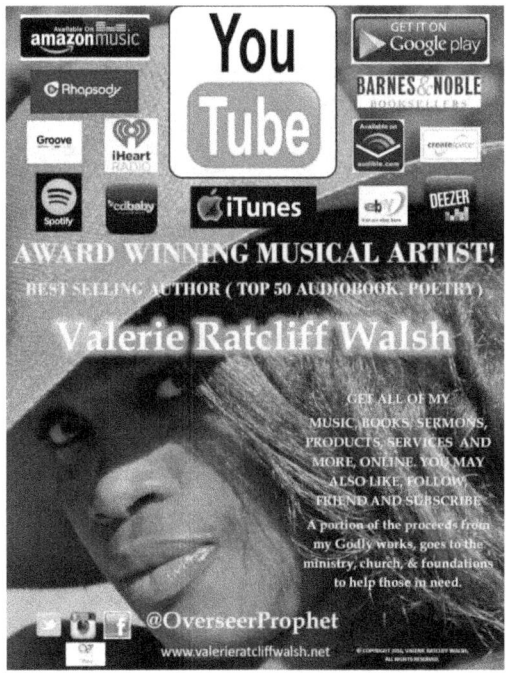

www.ingramcontent.com/pod-product-compliance
Lightning Source LLC
Chambersburg PA
CBHW061941280526
45787CB00004B/1678